A Comprehensive Couple's Guide To Oral Sex

Learn To Communicate & Satisfy

Overuntiy Publications

Copyright Notice

Copyright © Overunity Publications 2011. All rights reserved. None of the materials in this publication may be used, reproduced or transmitted, in whole or in part, in any form or by any means, electronic or mechanical, including photocopying, recording or the use of any information storage and retrieval system, without permission in writing from the publisher. To request such permission and for further inquiries, contact Overunity Publications at contact@overunitypublications.com

First Edition: 2011

ISBN 978-1468024197

Trademark Disclaimer

Product names, logos, brands, URLs, web site links, and other trademarks featured or referred to within this publication or within any supplemental or related materials are the property of their respective trademark holders. These trademark holders are not affiliated with the author or publisher and the trademark holders do not sponsor or endorse our materials.

Copyright Acknowledgment

Photographs attributed to a third party are the property of such third party and are used here by permission. All such attributed photographs are subject to the copyright claims of each respective owner.

Legal Disclaimer
Although the author and the publisher believe that the included information is accurate and useful, nothing contained in this publication can be considered professional advice on any legal or accounting matter. You must consult a licensed attorney or accountant if you want professional advice that is appropriate to your particular situation.

Author's Forward

Oral sex is one of my favorite intimate activities. There is a certain magic that exists between two partners engaged in oral sex, fellatio or cunnilingus, that just does not exist anywhere else in the sexual pantheon. Honestly, many times, in my life I have felt that oral sex is even more intimate than actual sexual intercourse. I love to go down on my committed partners, however, oral sex is something I would never consider with casual partners or one night stands. The magic is just missing. I'm sure many of my readers would agree. Many of my friends have been to prostitutes and not one of them has gone down on them. Hopefully, these empirical facts will help to put things in perspective. Oral sex is an act that truly reaches its zenith between two loving partners.

However, through my own research, I know that this act is too often ignored to the unsatisfaction of one or both partners in the couple. I hear one of two complaints frequently. The first is that oral sex is not even present in a relationship. One or both of the partners simply won't do it. The other is that oral sex, when it happens, is bad, short and misguided.

There are two distinct problems here. The first of these is a technical problem. Learning how to have intercourse is pretty basic. In fact, the lay it out for you in school. Oral sex, on the other hand is not so straightforward. This requires skills that they don't teach you in health class. You have to pick it up as you go along and all too often, people just don't get the instruction that
they need to truly blossom at the art.

Dealing with this, very surmountable, problem is the first aim of this book. The two chapters (originally published as separate books) will take both of the lovers through a very technical, easy to understand and follow class on both fellatio and cunnilingus. Once you have read through these pages, and given the techniques described a try, I am sure you will quickly become proficient at pleasing each other.

The other problem that this book is designed to address, is the communication gap that so often exists between partners where oral sex is concerned. The main source of this absence of talk seems to come from a fear that a person is no good at oral sex and is afraid of criticism. Well, working thorough these chapters, together, and reading the material, together, will quickly help to get you talking on the subject. Neither one of you should be afraid to point out something that you think that you would like to have done to you, or that you would like to try with your partner. Conversely, hopefully as you read these pages, you will encounter information that will make you ask questions and nourish a dialog. One way or the other, I am confident that the two of you will soon be building bridges to oral sex and not walls.

I wish you all the luck in the world.

Chapter 1
For Him
The Secret Art Of Eating Pussy
Tips & Tricks To Please Her Every Time

Eating a woman's pussy is one of the greatest sexual acts you can perform. It is at the same time intimate and incredibly sexual. You are literally making out with her pussy. At the same time that your head is buried between her thighs, you can feel the subtle convulsions of her body, her breath deepen and shorten and you can feel the arching of her back as she actually grinds her vulva into your face to heighten her own arousal. If you do it right, and you have a good partner in the woman, the experience is intense, unforgettable and at times - explosive.

There is a big "but", however. The sad truth is there are a lot of men out there who are so completely intimidated by this sexual act that they skip it altogether. Add them to the men who think they are great pussy eaters and aren't and you have a lot of men who just disappoint when they start going down on her. This document is designed to help deal with this problem. It is in effect, a little love letter to all those lovely pussies out there that I may never get to eat and a thank you to all those I have.

Now, let's get the cards on the table right now. When I first went down on a woman when I was sixteen, it was a dismal experience. Years of hardcore pornography mixed with my own adolescent exuberance made for one shabby performance. I didn't know where anything was, so I just licked everything and anything I could. I thought she would start to cum instantly, and was intimidated when she didn't. I tried to jam my whole hand inside of her in the hopes that I could find her g-spot. Add all that to the fact that I was terrified at my first close encounter with a pussy, and...well, you get the idea. No orgasm. Bad time. Disappointment was all around. It was just not good.

Replicate that miserable encounter with subtle variations for half a decade more, and you get a pretty good idea of my pussy eating background up until my early twenties. Pretty sad. The good thing was that I was so concerned with my own orgasm and indifferent to my partners, that it really didn't bother me. If I had actually stopped and thought, it would have, but I didn't. Then, everything changed.

I was engaged in some half assed pussy eating with a woman who must have just been fed up with men like me lacklusterly licking that garden of pleasure between her thighs. She actually told me to stop. I really think she had just had enough. She told me I was bad and what I was doing was just awful. She ended our little "romantic" encounter then and there. I was left with a hugely bruised ego and a raging hardon. Unfortunately her chiding had depressed me too much even to masturbate. It was a bad night.

It was a bad night, but as I look back now, I find that it was actually a pussy eating blessing in disguise. That pissed of woman with the girl equivalent of blue balls who was filled with disappointment actually opened my eyes and made me learn what I was actually doing wrong and what I needed to do right. She made it possible for me to actually pleasure the women in my life and to actually care about their experiences in the bedroom.

As I learned, a woman whose pussy has been eaten to three orgasms is a much more giving lover. Much more giving indeed. Add to that, the fact that when a woman knows you are going to take care of her needs before your own, she will want to make love with you more. Add to that the fact that when a woman can trust you with her pussy that she will open up sexually to you. Well – you get the picture. When you are good at eating pussy and the women in your life know it, you get more sex and better sex. I might also add that really pleasing a woman to the point that her thighs are convulsively shaking is a huge ego boost. It makes me feel even better than when I cum.

Let's Talk A Little Biology

A lot of people out there think that only lesbians know how to eat pussy really well. Well, this is true, as a general rule. They own the equipment and know a pussy well. This does give them an edge when it comes to eating pussy. However, as a man, you are not far behind.

You may or not know this, but every person starts out as a female embryo. Up to a point in development, we all have the same parts. At a certain point, however, hormones, cause these parts to differentiate and become male or female. A clitoris elongates and widens and becomes a penis. Vaginal lips develop into the scrotum. That's why you have that seam going down the middle. The passage through which a boy's testicles descend is really just a modified vagina. Mother nature is one weird and mad scientist.

Now don't go and freak out and suddenly wonder over whether you are a man or a woman. It's just a biological fact, and it can help to make you a great pussy eater. You see you actually have a pretty good idea of what feels good on your own genitals, and this gives you a pretty good idea (as a man) of what feels good to a woman as well. Our parts are different, but they are pretty similar.

Let's talk example to help clarify this point. Imagine you are getting a blowjob. Now, what do you want your partner to do? Do you want her to focus on your balls? Should she just lick away down there until all that ball licking makes you cum? Hell no. This isn't going to do anything towards you cumming. You don't want her just licking up and down the shaft of your penis either. This is nice, but you aren't going to orgasm from that either. In fact, all of this extra attention can be great, it can feel really good, but in the end, you want her to focus on the head of your penis while giving attention to all those other areas too. Well, women are exactly the same. They want you to focus your attention on their clitoris, while at the same time paying attention to all those other parts, in a lesser manner. That is the first secret right there. In the end, it's all about the clit. Focus your attention there.

Assume The Right Position

When I was first privileged enough to go down on a woman, I was young and dumb. I had seen a lot of porno movies and assumed that a woman could cum in any position, at any angle, from the slightest touch of my tongue. I couldn't come that way, but I assumed that the fairer sex had something I didn't. Well, turns out I was wrong there too.

You can eat a woman's pussy in any number of positions. You can get behind her when she is all fours (one of my favorites), you can have her sit on your face, or you can 69. Now, while she **CAN** come in any of these positions, the truth is that she probably won't. In order to orgasm, a woman must be comfortable and these positions are often too demanding for her physically and serve to distract. They are great for foreplay and for getting things wet. The thrill of these acts is good too. However, to really make a woman cum you need to have her on her back with her legs spread. This is your go-to, workhorse position. It just works. Remember that.

Admit You're Lost And Read The Damn Map

You need to be familiar with female anatomy if you can ever hope to be good at eating pussy. This is an absolutely critical part of your training and you need to spend some time getting to know what everything is and where you can find it. Most importantly, you need to know that a woman's pussy encompasses everything in the diagram above and all of it is sensitive. You can give her pleasure many different way through her many different parts and a good lover will know how.

Let's get started in this crash course of woman's anatomy.

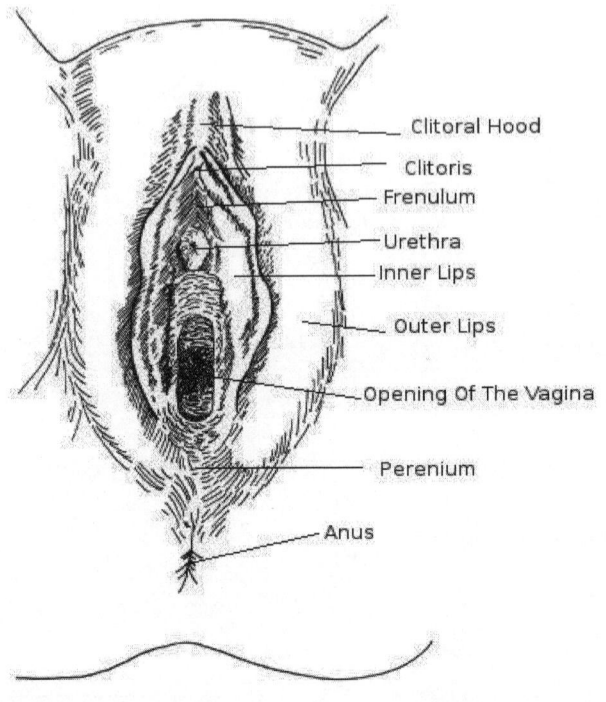

Start at the top of the diagram and we will work our way down. At the very top of her vagina, you will find her clitoris. This is the most famous tourist destination in a woman's pussy, and you should pay a lot of attention to this little organ. Now, remember, that a man's penis is simply a modified clitoris, or conversely, a clitoris is just a tiny penis. They are built along very similar lines. There is a tremendous amount of nerve endings in both. They are, however, much more concentrated in the clitoris. Stimulation of these nerves in both sexes are what gives everyone an orgasm. In men it results in ejaculation, in women, contractions of her vaginal muscles. In both sexes it feels great. The clitoris even swells when a woman is sexually excited just like the penis in men.

Now most men think the clitoris is really just a tiny button that they need to push. This is absolutely wrong. The clitoris is actually extends back and up on the woman's pussy and is protected by a layer of skin that can be pulled back. This skin is often called the clitoral hood and serves the same purpose as a foreskin on men, in that it protects the sensitive tissue. By placing your hand just above the woman's pussy (she is lying on her back with her legs spread) and gently pulling upward you can actually expose more of the clitoris. This exposes more nerve endings to your sucking and licking. Some women enjoy this and others will find it too intense.

Below the clitoris and inside the vaginal lips, above the urethra, you will find the vaginal frenulum. This is a soft, tender patch of skin that most people don't pay any attention to. This is a great area to stroke (after you have wet your finger with saliva). This is a stimulating act that will not lead to orgasm, however, it will very much heighten her arousal. That is a great secret right there.

The vaginal lips are another set of major features in the pussy that you need to be familiar with. There are two sets. The first is the labia majora. These are the lips that are often called camel toes. They are well developed and often covered with hair. The purpose of these lips are to protect all the delicate and tender bits immediately surrounding the vagina. It is by no means uncommon for you to need to spread these lips slightly with your fingers or tongue to gain access to the pussy itself. However, these are great for foreplay. One of my favorite subtly arousing techniques to to stroke the labia majora with my index and ring finger up and down. Do this very slightly so that your fingers are almost just tickling this area. As a more advanced technique, you can also **<u>GENTLY</u>** pinch the whole vaginal area between your thumb and the first knuckle of your index finger. Once you have done this, you can slowly move her whole pussy up (towards her clitoris) and down (towards her anus). This feels great over the whole pussy, and again, heightens the sense of arousal. Start your movements small and keep eye contact with her while you are doing this. This will increase your emotional connection and at the same time tune you into how she is enjoying the stimulation.

Inside the outer lips of the pussy (labia majora) you will find another set of lips. These are the labia minora or inner lips. These folds of tissue are immediately on the sides of the vaginal opening itself. These are very sensitive but they are also delicate. She will respond well to stimulation in this area, however, just like the clitoris, start softly and work up the pressure while you pay attention to her body movements. You don't want to hurt anything. The inner lips are also your guide to the clitoris itself. The clitoris is usually (not all women have the same pussy) located just below where the inner lips join at the top of the pussy. You can almost always follow them with your tongue or finger and they will lead you where you want to go.

The vaginal opening is contained inside her inner lips. This is where your penis goes during intercourse (I'm really hoping you already knew that). However, it can play a huge role in oral sex as well. However, you should really not spend a lot of time here with your mouth. There are nerve endings in the vagina for sure, however, you are really best inserting your fingers or a dildo in this area. (We'll talk more about this later.) Women love to have the feeling of being filled and simply inserting a finger or two will greatly enhance the oral sex. However, your mouth should spend most of its time either teasing the lips or stimulating her clitoris.

Below her vagina you will find her perenium. This is simple a patch of skin that divides her pussy from her anus. This is definitely a fun area to tease her with. You can put kisses here all day, however, there are no large amounts of nerve ends in this area.

Below her perenium is her anus. We will talk more about the anus later too.

Foreplay & Teasing

Men are very focused on the orgasm. We get so excited just watching a woman take her clothes off that we can't wait to cum. In doing so, we often cut our bedroom fun short. A man looking to become the kind of man that women brag about having been the lover of; needs to change this behavior. He needs to savor the non-intercourse parts of the sexual act and surrender to the soft touches and the loving caresses and even the teasing nips and licks that are part of the world of foreplay. This is nowhere more true than in giving oral sex to a woman.

To be good at the secret art of pussy eating, you need to excite the woman and make her feel desired. She needs to know that you are drinking in her scents, sights and sounds and that you cannot wait to give her pleasure in the most intimate of ways. To communicate this to her, as well as to give her pussy time to lubricate and be ready for your tickling tongue, you should spend a good part (I mean like 20-30 minutes) of time focusing on everything that is not her pussy.

Kissing is a great go to for foreplay. It is intimate, but not overtly sexual. It creates a connection and closeness and is also arousing. A favorite past time of mine is kissing up and down my lover's body. Focus on those parts that don't get lots of attention. Armpits, backs of knees, soles of feet and the labium majora (see illustration) are almost always looked over. They are all very sensitive and the kissing and gentle stroking of all of them is pleasurable and exciting. Of course there are the usual areas as well. My personal favorites are the belly button, the neck, the flanks, butt, thighs and breasts. Once you have kissed and given attention to all of these areas (even teased) you are then ready to begin kissing inside her pussy. She will be wet, waiting and eager for you to begin pleasuring her clitoris.

Get It Wet!

STOP! Before you go diving into the garden of sensual delights that is a woman's pussy, you need to learn something they never taught me in high school health class.

This is that a woman's pussy is very wet, and sensitive. The introduction of something dry and rough like your finger (or the head of your cock for that matter) can cause unpleasant sensations. It can cause dryness and can chafe the delicate tissues that are in there. She may be wet, willing and able if you have followed my advice on teasing and foreplay, but that does not mean that you still shouldn't be a gentleman.

I like to first open her pussy with my finger, and before I do this (every time) I lick my finger. I mean really lick, make sure there is a good amount of saliva on there to really get it wet and slippery. Then, and only then, can you begin to gently caress her in her most tender and intimate of places. As a bit of added good measure, I will usually give her pussy a good few, wet licks, with a soft tongue, before I ever even contemplate opening it with my finger. Again, this is like cutting your nails. It is one of those subtle, yet important, considerations for her comfort that will take you from being an ordinary, boring lover to an extraordinary, tell all her girlfriends, lover. It's worth a moment of your time.

Your Nails

From my research with the fairer sex, this seems to be one of the most overlooked secrets to eating pussy really well. You see, men are sturdy and well built. Penises can take a lot of abuse and are designed for just that. While vaginas are designed to take a lot of abuse too, they are more sensitive and a sharpened nail corner can really make for some unpleasant, sudden sensations.

Now, I am not telling you to go out and get a manicure every day. That would just be silly. What I am telling you to do is go out and buy a pack of emery boards. These are those little sanding boards that you always see woman using. They're cheap, so don't give me any excuses. Also, you are using these to make your girl cum while you eat her pussy, so don't bother saying they're effeminate either.

Before any date, or anytime you think you are going to wind up making out with a woman's bikini zone, make sure you clip your nails and then sand the hell out of them with the emery board. Pay closest attention to the corners of the nails. This is where they get really sharp. Take all of these down and make sure they have a nice, soft, rounded feel. Trust me, your girl will love this attention to her needs and will most likely pay closer attention to yours.

To Suck Or Lick?

In pussy eating discussions (like this one) the question of whether you should suck or lick the clitoris comes up quite a bit. The answer to this question is going to depend largely on the woman you are with. I have been with women you wanted me to do nothing more than to suck on the clitoris. Others, whose clits I have tried to suck did not care for the sensation at all. The suction was almost too much for them and they preferred I use the flat of my tongue instead.

Honestly, I prefer to use a technique that incorporates both of these tactics into one and really offers you the best of both worlds.

Get in front of a mirror and pay close attention to the steps that I am going to give you. Here is what you do:

1. Open your mouth about one inch wide. Basically, just relax your jaw muscles and let your lower jaw drop. This should feel natural and relaxed.
2. Stick your tongue out slightly until the tip of your tongue touches the center of your lower lip. The tip of your tongue should also be relaxed and rounded. Do not put a point on the tip of your tongue. This is the clit's worst enemy.

This is your perfect pussy eating mouth posture. What you do is place your whole mouth over the clitoral area. The flat of your tongue is used to stimulate the clitoris itself from below and the mouth can be used to either hold of suck on the clitoris depending on the woman's preference. If you do start sucking, start soft!!! This is a lot more sensitive than the head of your penis and you need to be gentle and work up. Suck too hard, and you can even hurt her.

This picture is a little crude, but it does serve to illustrate what I am describing:

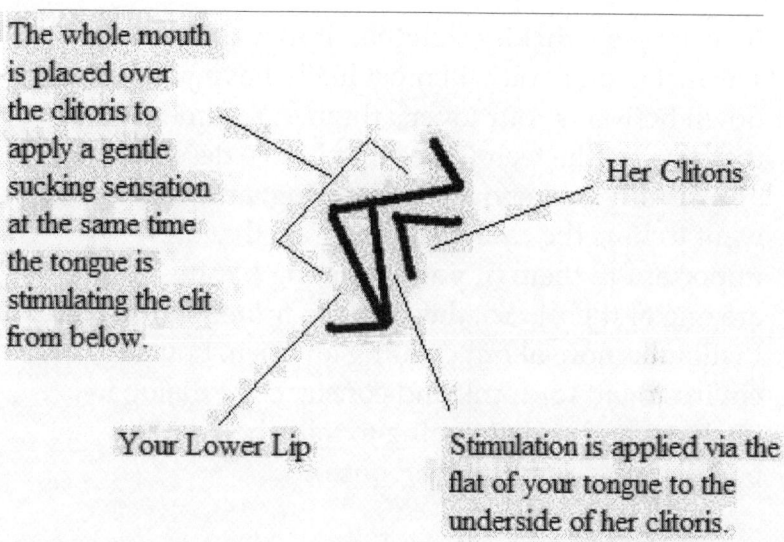

All of this will take a little coordination to master, but trust me, once you do, there is no telling how satisfied you can make your ladyfriends feel or how much they will appreciate your mastery of pussy eating secrets.

Taking Her Signals

The most important skill that you need develop to be a great pussy eater, is to be able to both perceive and to respond to the subtle signals that your lover will send you while you are between your thighs.

Now this is a trickier skill than it may first appear. The fact is that you will most likely have your head down between your lover's thighs. You may be focusing on the techniques that I have described to you. Lastly, women are very caring, and often don't want to hurt the feelings of the men that are important to them (if you are eating her pussy you are one of them). So, they tend to mute themselves. I will talk more about creating an open, honest environment for frank and constructive dialog in a bit, but for now, I am going to talk about subtle body signals and your responses.

It is possible for a woman to enjoy the pleasure you are giving her, while at them same time you are lost. Things can get confusing down there with all the hot and wet and writhing, and you may lose track of things. She may try to correct you. She will do this in one of two ways and you need to watch for these signals.

The first signal is that she will adjust her pelvis in order to bring the area she wants you to stimulate to the part of your mouth that's doing the stimulating. This is great. She is working with you, as a team, to give her an orgasm. This is exactly what you want. Relax and hold your head steady. The worst thing you can do in this situation is to move after what you think is her clitoris and instead just keep stimulating her labia. Women hate this. I know from my early years and nothing good is gong to come of it. So pay attention to the position of her pelvis when you are eating her pussy. If it moves suddenly, hold still and take her cues.

The other signal that she will offer is to grab your hair or head and redirect you. Again, this is exactly what you want. Direction from your partner as the two of you work to give her an orgasm. This signal is far less subtle and a lot of men take it as a criticism of their technique. Don't be a baby. She is is helping you and telling you what she wants to make her cum. This is rare and you need to grow up and take the direction like a good pussy eater. Trust me, once she is done cumming, it's going to be your turn and she will repay you in kind.

When I am eating a woman's pussy, I pay attention to all of these little motions and signals and I keep them in my mind. Later, as we bask in the afterglow of our orgasms and our sweaty bodies are wrapped together, I will often ask questions about these. I find after my lovers have cum that they are most honest and they will explain and offer criticism. This only adds to my skills and helps me to refine my technique to exactly what she wants. Remember, to be good at this, you need to take criticims and build it into your repertoire. Good lovers are not born, they are created through learning, discussion and experience.

KISS

A lot of men, when they fist come face to face with a pussy (a really wonderful moment indeed) have a tendency to go for the gold. They try to dazzle with rapid tongue twists and flicks. They try to impress her (the pussy's owner) with what they can do in the hopes that she will be seduced by the novel tricks that only they are privy too. They lick and suck anything and everything and probe their tongue in anywhere it can be received. These are all mistakes.

A woman does appreciate the attention to her areas, but again, think back and compare your cock and balls to a woman's pussy. What do you want? Do you want flash and trickery? Or do you want her to simply put the head in her mouth and suck while she works her hand up and down the shaft? Chances are that the second option is more appealing. Flash and tricks have their place in the foreplay aspect of pussy eating. However, when it comes time to get down to business, **K**eep **I**t **S**imple **S**tupid.

By this I mean, focus on the basics of stimulating her clitoris with your mouth, while at the same time giving her vagina a sense of being filled. That's it. That is a huge secret in mastering the art of pussy eating. Focus on those two things, and you are well on your way to making a lot of women's cheeks rosy and a lot of thighs shake.

Forget The G-Spot

The G-spot, or Grafenburg Spot, is supposed to be an area located inside a woman's vagina. Honestly, the g-spot falls into that category somewhere between fiction and reality. There is still a great deal of robust debate between physiologists as to whether or not it exists at all. That being said, some women do claim to be able to orgasm from the stimulation of a zone on the front wall of the vagina, about two inches inside.

OK, let's talk plainly here. Some women claim to be able to orgasm from the stimulation of a so called "G-spot". Some people have claimed to be abducted by aliens and to have seen the Loch Ness monster. Some people will claim just about anything. You are a man (most likely) and you are trying to make sense of a woman's erogenous zones, and honestly, the g-spot just confuses the matter. Unlike the clitoris, which has a male counterpart in the penis, the g-spot has no counterpart that would explain its existence. Additionally, there is not even proof of a super sensitive tissue like there is with the clitoris. I have spoken to women who even feel dysfunctional because they have never been able to find their g-spot during masturbation. OK. So they can't find it. That means that as a man while eating a woman's pussy, you have about 0% chance of finding it.

All of this controversy, and many men still go on a mythical quest to find the g-spot. Here is another pussy eating secret. Forget what all those magazines say. Don't bother with the g-spot. Don't even bother looking for it. Focus on her clitoris. We are all sure its real and direct clitoral stimulation is the best way to give a woman an orgasm.

Don't Talk!!!!

A lot of young men have learned to have sex and eat pussy by watching porno movies. It's a sad cultural commentary, but it's true. They think girls want them to pull out before they cum and do it all over their chests. They think girls will cum at their slightest touch and they think women want you to say encouraging things when they are eating their pussy. I know, I was one of these men. I also know now, that all of this is wrong.

When you are eating a woman's pussy, your mouth should be doing only one thing – eating pussy. Don't say anything. Common phrases to avoid are:

    1. Cum for me baby

2. Do you like that?
3. Are you going to cum?
4. Did you cum?

Just shut up. Don't say anything. When you talk you do one of or both of two bad things. First, you put pressure on them to perform (i.e. orgasm). Women don't cum when you put pressure on them to perform. Their orgasm has to come naturally. Talking and encouraging them is not helpful. Also, when you talk you are not stimulating their clit.

Have you ever had a girl stop giving you a blowjob right at that critical first second of orgasm? Everything goes to hell quickly and the orgasm fails to happen. This is a huge disappointment to you and you stopping sucking on their clit can do the same thing to a woman. Just don't!

Just Keep Going

You need to be patient when you are eating a woman's pussy, especially the first time. How long a woman takes to cum during oral sex depends on a lot of factors. She needs to know that you are into the act. That you are enjoying yourself. She needs to relax. She needs to be able to enjoy the physical stimulation and feel connected to her lover. All of this takes time.

One of the worst mistakes a man can make when a woman has chosen to let him make out with her pussy is to get impatient. He starts to worry that his technique is bad and asks "Is something wrong?". At this point, she is now under pressure and most likely will never relax enough to orgasm. Congratulations, you just killed her boner.

Instead, what you need to do is have faith in your technique and just keep going. Don't worry about time at all. Enjoy the act of eating her pussy for the act of eating her pussy and relax. Just get in there and eat it. Trust me.

Another point about "Just Keep Going" is you should never stop until the woman tells you to. That is another secret. **DO NOT STOP UNTIL TOLD TO DO SO.** If you stop before you are told to because you think that she just orgasmed, you may be wrong. You may interrupt her orgasm and ruin it. It happens to every man at some point in his life. He's just about to cum and then something happens to ruin it all. Maybe he falls off the bed or gets a cramp. Whatever it is, he gets right to that point, he's just about to explode and boom. Nothing. You can't even get back there and now you're frustrated that you can't cum at all. Don't do that to her.

The last reason you just keep going until she tells you to stop is that you may have gotten so good at eating her pussy from reading this that you are venturing into multiple orgasm territory. Women can cum more than once in quick succession. She may have completed one orgasm and her pussy muscles may be tightening in preparation for another, even bigger one, when you decide to stop. The same thing happens that I described above. Nothing good.

So, long story short. Get in there and start eating your woman's pussy and just don't stop until she tells you no matter what. You may be rewarded by her screaming out "STOP, I can't take it anymore!", while her legs are shaking and she's had four orgasms. Think what she'll tell her girlfriends then.

Shave Before

This is definitely the "duh" section of this book, but I am putting it in here because a lot of men are...well naive. A penis is meant to take a lot of punishment. You can have a woman bouncing up and down on that thing all day and it won't cause any damage. I have even whacked a thing or two with mine to no ill effect. A vagina is very different. There are a lot of sensitive tissues in there that get irritated very easily. Even a little bit of stubble can present a problem. So, be a gentleman and just shave thoroughly. She will appreciate it.

No Spicy Foods

This one is a little funny now, but at the time it was not a good experience. When I was nineteen or so, I took a woman out for Mexican food. We went to town and had a feast. I love spicy food so I loaded up all my tacos with plenty of the picante sauce.

Well, one thing lead to another and before long, I was eating her pussy. I was into it. She was into it. Well, then the capsicum that I had been eating started doing some not nice things to her pussy. I'm not talking third degree burns or anything, but I am talking irritation and the need for a cooling shower.

Now, famous inventors have failed many times before they finally perfected their invention and gave us things that we use everyday. This is how I look at my pussy eating technique at that point. This was an early failure that certainly taught me one way to **NOT** eat a woman's pussy. This doesn't mean that you can't take her out for something spicy. However, if you do, rinse your mouth with milk (half and half is even better) before you start kissing her most intimate and delicate of places. That's another true pussy eating secret.

Accept Not 100%

If you are reading this, you are a man who wants to eat the pussy the right way. That means that you care about the sexual pleasure of your partner(s). That means that you always want sex to finish after your girl has had an orgasms and everybody is glowing with post sex energy. Most likely you want that 100% of the time, and this usually means some pussy eating. Great.

Well, the truth is that nothing is 100%. Sometimes you can't cum when your girlfriend is giving you a blowjob. Maybe you have a big presentation tomorrow at work. Maybe you're just tired. It happens. It happens to them too. Sometimes a woman just wants to have sex and feel connected to you, but she's just not in the mood for oral sex. That's OK too. If you are reading this, you are a gentleman, and one of the pussy eating secrets that a gentleman needs to accept, is that it isn't perfect 100% of the time. Accept it. Move on and roll with it. It doesn't make you any less of a man or any less of a lover. I know from experience.

Communicating With Your Partner

Good pussy eating is not something that you do alone. It's like a dance. You need to have a good partner and work together or nothing interesting is going to happen. Without good communication, all the secrets that you have learned in this article are worthless. So talk to your partner.

Talking to your partner is the ultimate secret that I can pass on to you. You need to know what she likes. Don't be afraid to ask questions. Do not assume you are the expert concerning her body. She is and she can tell you everything that you need to know.

I always talk to my ladyfriend after I perform oral sex on them for the first time. I ask questions and I try to encourage honest answers. I always stress to them that I don't want them to worry about my feelings or ego and I certainly don't want them to fake it. I emphasize how much i love to eat their pussy and how much pleasure it gives me to please them. I encourage them to feel confident in telling me what to do when I am down there. Just bark out orders. I like that. This helps empower them and makes them feel like an enthusiastic participant in getting them off. This makes them more eager to participate in oral sex and it makes the oral sex better and their orgasms stronger.

Everything about pussy eating gets better when you have an open and continuing dialog with your partner and you foster honesty in your communication.

Basic Fingering

Fingering is a very important part of eating pussy well and it is a skill you are going to have to master. Fortunately, there is not a lot that you need to know to make you good at this skill.

First off, the reason that women like to be fingered while you are eating their pussy is that it adds to the sensation. You are stimulating their vagina with your finger at the same time that you are pleasuring their clit with your mouth. Unfortunately a lot of men do this wrong. Fingering is really like table salt, a little will go a long way and most men over do it. I am going to tell you how to do it just right.

First off, you should always start fingering with just one finger. Remember to get it wet first. Go ahead and just suck it for a second to make sure that there is plenty of saliva and it won't stick to or pull any of her delicate tissues. Next, find the opening to her vagina gently. Don't jam it in there. Slide your moistened fingertip up and down her inner lips until you find it. Slowly insert up to the first knuckle and then move your finger around in a circle. Doing this helps her to open up and makes sure that her vagina is wet enough for you to proceed. If she is not wet enough pause for a moment and help her out.

There are two ways that you can help to get her wet. You can first stimulate her clitoris for a few minutes. This will encourage her natural vaginal lubrication. You can also lick up and down her inner lips and vagina with a good amount of saliva. Then you use this saliva to help lubricate her vagina with the tip of your finger. I would recommend doing a combination of the two, although either one will work on its own. Once she is wet enough (I cannot emphasize how important her being lubricated is) you can proceed with inserting a finger all the way. Start with one again. Make sure she's wet and then move up to two fingers. In most cases, this is perfect. Don't go above two unless she tells you to.

Now, the mistake that most men make is that you are going to need to pull your finger in and out while you are eating her pussy. They think that they need to simulate a penis for her to feel anything. This is a big mistake. In fact, pounding away with your finger can be distracting to her and may actually ruin the pussy eating. There are two fingering methods that I will pass on to you here. Both feel great to her and are not distracting.

First, insert your two fingers (I prefer index and middle) all the way. Now, apply subtle, slow pressure into her vagina and then relax. This act will apply pressure to her vaginal opening and will give her a lot of the same sensation as she would get during intercourse. Next, you can tilt your fingers down in the direction of her anus. This applies pressure to the muscles inside of her vagina and again, simulates intercourse, without the need to bang away. Both of these techniques together make for the perfect fingering combination. Remember, slow subtle pressure, not fast in and out jack hammering.

It is also perfectly possible to eat your woman's pussy well without fingering. In fact, adding fingering is a complication that may be hard for you to keep track of when you first start eating her pussy. Trying to keep track of her clit while she is bucking her hips and fingering her at the same time may be overwhelming and confuse you. If you feel that you can't keep track of everything at first, ditch the fingering and instead focus on just stimulating her clit. That is the important part. I have done that plenty of times and everything usually works out just fine. Once you feel more confident with her body and you have the rhythm of things down, you can always take it up a notch by reintroducing fingering.

Toys

You are more than welcome to master the art of eating pussy without toys. Honestly, I tend to prefer to keep things manual, and impromptu pussy eating does not allow me to grab a toy anyway. However, toys definitely have a place in this discussion and they definitely have a place in pussy eating.

There are two types of sex toys that you should consider having where eating your ladyfriend's pussy is concerned. The first is a small clitoral vibrator. The other useful sex toy is a silicone dildo.

There are a lot of vibrators out there. More than you could possible imagine. They all have their use and place, however for eating her pussy, all you really are going to need is a clitoral vibrator. A clitoral vibrator is a small, couple inches at most, that is used directly on her clitoris. Depending on the model, they can pulsate at single or multiple speeds, or even go through preset patterns.

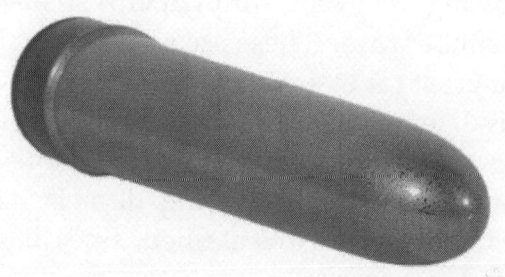

Now, if the vibrator is working on her clit, your tongue is not and then you are not really eating her pussy. Why do you need one then? Well, in some cases, you may not be able to finish her off with your mouth alone. Sometimes your jaw will get tired, or she will need more stimulation than your tongue can offer. Well, in that case, this little guy can act like a stand-in for you. You still get the intimacy of oral sex, however, she gets the intense stimulation that the industrial revolution has made possible. This is not a bad thing at all.

Now, dildos are another story. Dildos do not offer any vibrating. They are simply penis shaped silicone rubber toys. These are great for oral sex. They are great for inserting into her vagina while you stimulate her clitoris with your mouth. This gives her the sensation of being filled, more so than fingering can. As with fingering, don't jack hammer away. She just wants to feel filled. She doesn't need any ramming going on.

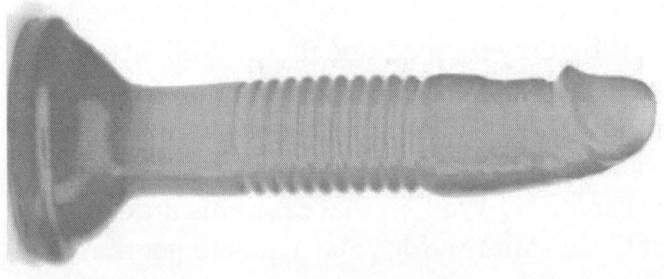

The size of the dildo is important. Some of these toys can be as big around as a soda can. You don't need that. As a good rule of thumb, get a dildo that is just a little smaller than your penis. This will definitely fill her up, however, you won't be outshined by a piece of rubber.

Leave Her Ass Alone...At First

A lot of men assume that just because a woman is letting them eat her pussy, that she is just dying to have them play with her ass too. Well, sorry to burst your bubble, but that just isn't the case. Yes, there are some women out there who do like attention there, however, I have certainly found them to be in the minority.

Do yourself and your woman a favor. Don't go for her ass the first time without having talked about it. If you go there and it isn't OK, you probably will ruin the pussy eating (if you even get to finish) and you may not be asked back between her thighs. If you are one of those men who has an ass fetish (nothing wrong with that) bring it up once you have been having regular sex for a while. That's when its OK, and there's no harm in asking.

Where Her Mind Is

To be a good pussy eater, you are going to need to be empathetic to your woman and understand just how personal it is to let someone bury their face between your thighs. In many cases I have known women who would happily have intercourse with someone over having them eat their pussy, simply because their confidence did not permit it.

Women worry a lot about their pussies. They are often thinking questions like:

1. Does my pussy smell?
2. Is my pussy weird looking?
3. Is my pubic hair OK?

This is a major self confidence issue for many women and it is going to be up to you to convince her that you are absolutely wild over her pussy. I do this lots of ways. I get in there and niff and savor. I pass lots of compliments (that are true of course) about their pussies. I tell them how beautiful they are and how good they smell and taste. I tell them how much I am enjoying going down on them and I try to go down on them any chance I get. Lots of foreplay helps too. This will help her relax and surrender to them moment and the pleasure.

Essentially, you need to do everything you can to reassure your woman that what is between her legs is not only attractive to you, but that you can't wait to get it in your mouth. After a while she will believe you and this makes the oral sex even better, but in the beginning, you need to do a lot to reassure her. You should also avoid common pitfalls like suggesting she take a shower before you eat her pussy. This is just a huge hit to her ego and I have known a few men who fell into this one. Just don't! Let her be the judge on that. If you are a gentleman who is truly interested in pleasuring your woman, you will do like me and jump on any chance she gives you to eat her pussy, anytime!

Bask In The After Glow

Once her legs are trembling from all the orgasms you have given her and her clit is so sensitive that she can't even bear your touch, you should probably give her pussy a break. This is a great time to make her feel close and connected to you. She has just let you perform the most intimate of all sex acts and she is open to you. Get close and hold her. Snuggle. Kiss. Enjoy each others company. Don't talk too much, just listen to each other and feel connected. Often, this will lead to intercourse, and post pussy eating intercourse is some of the best you will ever have. You will be excited from having made out with her pussy and she will feel strongly connected to you and her pussy is alive with sensation. Don't initiate the intercourse. Be a gentleman. Let her rest for a moment. If she wants it, she will let you know. Just watch for the signs.

I have taught you the basic skills that you are going to need to become a master pussy eater. Work hard at this skill. Women pay lip service to pussy eating, but they all love it. A man who is both open and eager to perform this skill, as well as one who actually knows what he is doing is rare. Most men just don't make the cut. You have taken the first step in the path that leads away from that group.

You must take other steps. You are going to need to get out there and eat some pussy. You are going to need to work hard to train yourself to notice all those subtle signals I talked about. You are going to need to master her anatomy and know how she likes to be touched. However, you are on your way to becoming the kind of lover that women really only dream of. Congratulations.

Chapter 2
For Her
The Secret Art Of The Blowjob

Tips & Tricks To Please Him Every Time

Last year I wrote a book dedicated to the secret art of pussy eating (The Secret Art Of Eating Pussy: Tips & Tricks To Please Her Every Time ISBN 978-1463655631). It was well received. However, the release of that book has resulted in a number of communications asking me to provide a similarly written guide to those who are out there trying to please a man orally.

At first I thought it odd. Women asking a man to teach them to suck cock. It honestly seemed like a book that a woman should write. Then I thought about it. Most men have trouble openly discussing topics like this and have even more trouble explaining their ideas clearly and concisely. Often they are afraid of critiquing the blowjob performances of their lovers. They are often afraid of hurting their feelings. What I realized was happening was these women were asking for my help to make their sex lives more fulfilling and richer. Well, I am never one to shrink from a challenge. So, I sat down, thought a lot, and toiled a fair amount writing this little how to for all those out there looking to learn the secrets of a good blowjob.

I have also done an exhaustive empirical study into the subject of blowjobs from the point of view of both sexes. I'm not going to lie, I had to buy a lot of pitchers of beer and shots to get some of those girls and more of the guys to open up on the subject. However, they did. They shared many, many, juicy and intimate details about the subject. Also, my conversations have really run the gamut from man on man blowjobs, to woman on man blow jobs, to man and woman blowjobs...well, you get the point. I have hit all the bases.

So in essence, I have been the recipient and provider of a lot of oral sex and I have talked with my wide and varying peer group to get a true, intimate understanding of the blowjob from every perspective. The distillation of that essence is this work. It is my sincere hope, that through the study of this work, you will learn how to amaze, wow, tantalize and orally ravish the luck man in your life. Let's get started!

A Discussion Of Male Anatomy

In order to be able to successfully give a blowjob to a man, you need to have a basic understanding of a man's penis. When I wrote about eating pussy, I included a similar discussion. This is no different. However, a person interested in giving a blowjob does have one advantage over someone wanting to eat pussy. The vagina is a touch on the secretive side. Many of her secrets are hidden inside lips and folds of skin. With the penis, everything is very out in the open.

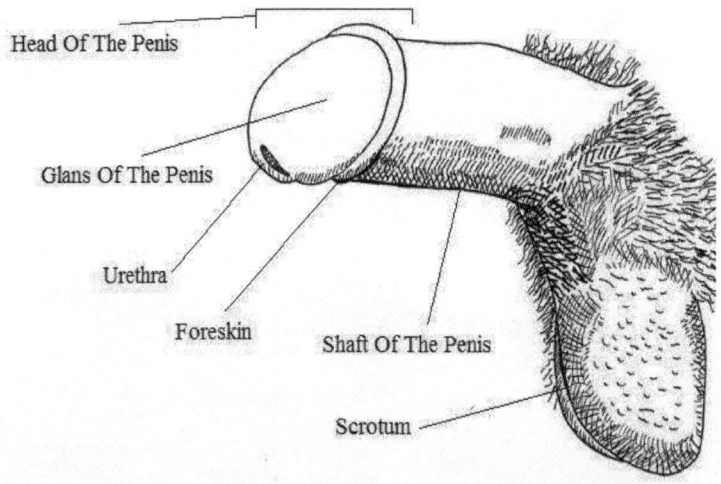

Obviously the penis itself is most prominent. However, I do want to highlight a few aspects of the penis that will be helpful to you in your quest to master the art of the blowjob. The penis is actually made up of several parts and they differ in sensitivity and how you stimulate them.

At the very tip of the penis, you will find the opening of the man's urethra. This is where he will ejaculate from. This opening is at the very center of what is often called the glans of the penis. The man is most sensitive at this point. The highest concentration of nerves on the penis are found here. This means this is where you can stimulate him the most. As you move out from the opening of his urethra along the skin of the "helmet" of his penis, this concentration of nerves decreases rapidly. By the time you reach the shaft of his penis, the sensitivity has fallen sharply. When you are stimulating a penis with your mouth, you really only need to focus on the "helmet" of his penis for this reason. This is the most pleasure sensitive area of his whole body.

As a way to help put everything in context, I want to remind the reader about a fact of biology. When a human embryo is just beginning to develop, male and female embryos are essentially identical. If everything continues on uninterrupted, the embryo will develop female. However, if the right hormones are in place, the embryo will undergo a few modifications and turn male. In this process, the tissues that would normally form the clitoris elongates and develops and turns into a penis. The tissue that would form vaginal lips instead seal up and form his scrotum. That's why that seam runs up the middle of it.

Think of it this way and you will do very well. The same nerves that are present in your clitoris are the same nerves that are present in the glans of your lover's penis. The way you like your clitoris to be stimulated orally, is the same way that he wants his penis to be stimulated by your mouth.

I do want to pause for a moment and discuss foreskin. If your partner is not circumcised, it will be necessary for you to wrap your fingers around his penis and slowly push down towards his balls to reveal the tip of his penis. It is entirely possible that the entire tip of his penis is concealed by the foreskin when his penis is limp. This is where the term "snake in a sweater" comes from. If this is the case, do not be alarmed. Once he becomes hard and you apply the pressure to the foreskin I described above, the tip of his penis will be revealed and everything else is the same.

Continuing down the male anatomy, we next come to the shaft of the penis. This area is considerably less sensitive than the glans of his penis. Your mouth can be used in this area for playful licking and kissing, or even deep throating. However, it is not required here in order to give a good blowjob.

Below the shaft of the penis we come to the man's testicles. Now, here women are often stumped. I honestly can't blame them. The testicles and the scrotum are a bit of a mystery. Women know that men like attention here, however, they are often afraid of causing any harm. OK, here is the guiding principle surrounding the testicles. Just be gentle. Yes, men like attention to their balls. The enjoy it. However, you need to be gentle. You can kiss, lick, lightly suck or lightly caress. Support is good too. Cup them and hold them with your free hand. However, remember that roughly sucking or grabbing can quickly ruin the party. If you are ever unsure, start very, very gently and work your way up slowly. You will find the right attention for the man you are playing with quickly enough.

Below his balls you will find his perenium. This is often called the "taint". This particular area is not terribly sensitive, however, you can definitely give it some attention. If you don't want to go here, don't worry. You will can still give him an amazingly wonderful blowjob without ever paying this area any attention.

Lastly, we come to his anus. It is true that some men like to have their anus played with during a blowjob. It can be kissed, licked or even fingered. However, many women are uncomfortable with this. If you are, don't give it a second thought. What I said about the "taint" is just as true here. However, if you are one of those people who really wants to play with an anus (I can be one of them from time to time to), you need to leave it alone until you have talked with your partner. This is one of those areas where communication is key. You need to talk and see what they think. A surprise anus raid is never something that should happen. Both partners need to be into it and excited by it, or it shouldn't happen.

Now that we are on the same page concerning the important points of a man's anatomy, we can get down to our technical discussion of blowjobs. Let's move on.

Communication Is Still Key

I stressed this in my book on pussy eating and I want to stress this again in this work. The best way to achieve a successful environment for passionate, erotic, hot, mind blowing oral sex is through communication. I can and will teach you a lot of techniques in this book, however, only through communication can you learn how your particular partner likes them to be applied.

You need to be able to talk to him, and you need to talk to him about your blowjobs. Now, don't go and take any criticism as meaning you are a poor cock sucker. On the contrary! The fact that you know that every man is different and that only through talking to him can you learn how to blow him perfectly, already makes you a better blowjobber than most of the women out there.

I would recommend three ways that you can communicate about his enjoyment and your technique. If you are normally shy, don't be. Every man loves talking about blowjobs.

First, you can do a pregame conversation. This is when you ask what he likes before you have his throbbing member staring you in the face. Ask him what was the best blowjob he ever had. Ask him what he likes to have done. This alone will be more than enough to start getting blood flowing to his crotch. You can gain a lot of insight about his particular pleasure triggers from this conversation.

The next opportunity to engage in communication is during the blowjob itself. Now, in this situation, you are not going to be able to carry on an extensive deep dialog. If you are talking a a lot during a blowjob, I'm sorry, but you're doing it wrong. Limit yourself to the simple question; "Do you like that?". Look him in the eye when you say it and see how he reacts. Is he excited and enthusiastic? If he is, you are on the right track. Now, don't go and ask this every two seconds. That will make him feel like you are interrogating him. Limit yourself to asking this question three times. Other than that, you will need to rely on his body movements to see if he is enjoying what you are doing. We will talk about that more later.

The last opportunity you will have to talk to your man about your blowjob performance is after the blowjob is over. The best time is while he is basking in the afterglow and is still a little drunk from the orgasm you just gave him with your mouth. Ask him if he liked it. Ask him what his favorite part was. Most likely his answers will be short and to the point, but they will be honest.

The Basic Blowjob Technique

When I wrote "The Secret Art Of Eating Pussy: Tips & Tricks To Please Her Every Time", I advised the reader of that book to forget about all the bells and whistles and simply focus on stimulating the clitoris in a basic manner. All to often in our lives we seek to complicate the simple and in doing so lose sight of our goal. The same is true with blowjobs.

The primary goal of the blowjob is simply to use your mouth to make the man orgasm. That's it. To do that, all you need to do is to stimulate the glans of his penis with your mouth, while at the same time, stimulating the shaft of the penis with your hand. That's it! Congratulations, you just learned the first secret to giving really good head. Keep that simple goal in mind and the men in your life will think you are amazing at giving oral sex in no time.

Now, there are some details to work out to give this basic blowjob. First, you need to focus on body positioning. You can really suck a cock in more ways than I could possibly describe. You can come at it from an almost infinite number of ways. However, just like there is a basic pussy eating position, there is a basic blow job position as well.

The easiest way to give a basic blowjob is to have your lover lie down on the bed. You can have them stand, but honestly, he can stumble when he's cumming and your knees can get sore. A bed fixes both of these problems. Have him spread his legs and you get between them facing him. This position is also good, because when you put his penis in your mouth, your tongue will be along the bottom of his glans. This will increase stimulation.

You should be up on your knees. You are going to be using your hands here, so you cannot rely on them to support your body. You arms should be able to have full freedom of motion. That being said, take hold of his penis with your hand (for brevity, I am assuming he's already erect). Your hand should be holding his penis like you would a bottle of beer. Your thumb should be on the same side that you are and the outside of your pinky should be resting on his body, just where his penis attaches.

Now, you are going to stroke his penis with your hand. Don't worry, we're going to get your mouth involved, but we have to build to that. Gently grasp his penis and move your hand up it. When he is hard, you will feel the skin slide over the muscle in his penis. This is perfect. Gently, at first, slide your hand up the shaft of the penis until the edge of your index finger touches the start of the helmet of his penis. Once you have hit that point, do the opposite and slide your hand back down until your pinky touches his body. This is the basic blowjob hand motion.

Now, you will notice that the basic blowjob hand motion does nothing for the tip of his penis. You may be wondering why this is, since we have already talked about how many nerves are there and how stimulated that little patch of skin can get. Well, have no fear, that is where your mouth comes in.

Go ahead and place the tip of his penis in your mouth. All you really need in there is the helmet of the penis. That is really all that is necessary for giving a good, basic blowjob. Hold in in your mouth and slowly slide your tongue from side to side on the underside of the tip of his cock. Suck in ever so slightly to create just the faintest hint of pressure. You do not need to compete with the vacuum cleaner. Think gentle pressure only. This is the basic blowjob mouth motion.

The goal of the basic blowjob is to combine the basic blowjob hand motion with the basic blowjob mouth motion. The two together make the overall experience so much more pleasurable than either one could ever be on it own. Go ahead and try it at this point if you can. Now, don't start to fast with your hand or you will be hitting yourself in the face. Start slowly and get the rhythm down. It won't take long. Actually, starting slow in the beginning will help to heighten his arousal. Speed up when you are more comfortable and really go to town when he shouts out "I'm going to cum. Don't Stop!".

Congratulations. You have just learned how to perform a basic blowjob. That forms the core of this book. Everything else that we will discuss adds to and enhances this concept. However, trust me, with this information alone, you are perfectly capable of pleasing any man in your life.

Lube, Lube, Lube

When you are stroking the shaft of his penis at the same time that you have the tip in your mouth, you are going to be applying some friction. This is good. This is what is stimulating him and what will ultimately lead to his orgasm. However, just like friction in your vagina, lubrication helps to make everything work smoothly and pleasurably.

Now, I am not telling you to squirt a water based lube all over his junk. This will just cause a sticky mess and wind up in your mouth. You don't need or want this to occur. Instead, rely on your saliva to keep everything lubricated.

What you need to do is literally drool on his cock as you are sucking it. Don't worry one second that he will be upset that you are drooling all over his cock. In fact, he will probably really get off on it. Some of the best blowjobs I have ever had are the sloppiest, drooliest ones. The saliva keeps everything lubricated until I am orgasming.

As a twist to the whole drooling on his cock concept while you are sucking and stroking it, you can always spit on his dick to keep it lubed. Spitting on it has the same lubricating effect that discreetly drooling on it does with one added advantage. He will see it and hear it. The act of spitting on his cock will appeal very much to almost any man out there. Think of it as a show woman's way of keeping everything good and wet. You achieve a necessary function at the same time you heighten his arousal. Whatever you choose to do, just keep his cock well lubricated while you are stroking it.

Don't Stop Until Your Told To

One of the worst things that any woman can do while giving a blowjob is to stop prematurely. This can have disastrous results. Imagine the last time that you got oral sex and had an orgasm. You might be smiling with reminiscences. Well, now try and imagine your lover stopping right at that critical moment that your orgasm was peaking. Boom! All of a sudden all of the stimulation is gone. That wonderful orgasm that had been building for what seemed like forever vanishes. Worst of all, at that point, there is no way to get it back. You've missed it like a bus on a rainy day and you're stuck out in the cold. Now you've got sexual frustration instead of orgasmic afterglow.

Well, men and women are not really that different and our orgasms are based on similar processes in our bodies. When he begins to ejaculate his orgasm is only just beginning to peak. Trust me, the first drop of semen does not mean his orgasm is over. It is only starting. What he needs to truly climax at that moment is the same consistent stimulation that you have applied up to this point. Stopping prematurely, when you feel the first spurt of semen, will just ruin his orgasm.

This means two things. First, it means that you are going to have to deal with his semen one way or another. I will talk about the options that you have at your disposal later on. However, you need to plan this out before your mouth starts filling with semen. Next, it means that in order to truly give a fantastic, amazing blowjob, you are going to need to continue your mouth work until he has finished his orgasm. Just as your clitoris becomes super sensitive after orgasm, the tip of his penis will too. At a certain point it is so sensitive that he will not be able to tolerate your sucking and will tell you to stop. Either that, or his cock will begin to go limp. Those are the two signs that you have that it is safe to stop. Either he will tell you or his cock will. Either way, wait til then.

Cumming In The Mouth...Let's Talk

A lot of women out there are intimidated by the thought of having their lover cum in their mouths. As such, they do one of two things.

The first thing that often occurs when a woman is afraid of getting some semen in her mouth, is that she just flat out refuses to give her lover oral sex. Now, of course this is her prerogative, however, in doing so she is denying her lover a pleasurable and very intimate form of sex and she is missing out on all the positive rewards of performing a blowjob. Performing a blowjob successfully makes you feel attractive, sexy, appreciated and the pure act of giving pleasure to your lover is pleasurable to you. Obviously, missing out on all this is not good.

The other thing that a woman with a semen phobia is going to do is give a half assed blowjob and stop the oral stimulation about halfway through. Then she will usually manually stimulate her lover until he cums all over her. She is fine with this, she just doesn't want to get it in her mouth. This can be fine, but honestly, it is going to be a pretty unimpressive blowjob.

He wants to cum in your mouth. There, I said it. You just need to accept it. If you are going to become a blowjob goddess, which is the aim of this book, you are just going to have to come to grips with the fact that you are going to need to let your lover cum in your mouth. It may be awkward at first. So is eating oysters, however, you will get used to it and probably, in the long run learn to enjoy it.

Let me explain why he wants to cum in your mouth in a manner that you can most likely relate to. I am going to assume that you, as a woman, have received oral sex before and orgasm ed from it. Close your eyes and imagine the warm wet sensation of your lovers mouth all over your pussy. It feels great. You are starting to build towards orgasm and you can feel all those little tremors in your thighs starting to shoot off. You can't want. You get closer and closer as the person between your thighs pleasures you in perfect rhythm with your own movements. Then...they stop and start trying to give you an orgasm with just their fingers. The magic will get broken. You may be able to get there eventually, but now, everything is different. You are a little frustrated and you have to start all over.

That scenario is exactly what is happening when you take his penis out of your mouth and switch to giving him a handjob. He may get there eventually, but usually it will be frustrating and the magic is gone.

Instead, just plan on letting him cum in your mouth. You don't have to swallow anything and I will give you several techniques to deal with the semen.

Overcoming The Fear Of Ejaculation

The first point that needs to be addressed before you are comfortable dealing with semen in your mouth is we need to get you over the fear of him cumming in your mouth. A lot of women are afraid of this. There is nothing wrong with that fear. It is a little odd and the act is foreign. Of course they have all heard horror stories from their friends about choking and what not. No one likes water going down their throat when they are swimming and semen in your throat is pretty much the same thing.

As a rule, when he is about to cum, you should just have the tip of his penis in your mouth. This will help you to control the ejaculation and it will also reduce the chance of any semen going down your windpipe. This is to be avoided, as it will prompt a violent coughing fit.

It is not at all unreasonable to ask your lover to tell you when they are getting close to orgasm. This opens the channels of communication and serve three very good purposes. The first purpose is that you will not be caught with a mouthful of semen while you are unprepared. You can get ready for it and deal with it accordingly when it happens. Secondly, just like when someone is eating your pussy, you don't want things to change when he is very close to orgasm anyway. Calling out that he is about to cum will help you keep the rhythm steady and ensure that his orgasm occurs without any frustrating interruptions. The last purpose that this serves is to build trust between a couple. You will be able to trust that he is not going to cum in your mouth without telling you. This will help you relax and really begin to enjoy giving him pleasure and feeling sexy and empowered in return.

Before you begin to give him a blowjob, ask him to tell you when he is about to cum. Trust me, he will be more than happy to accommodate your request if it means he gets a blowjob and gets to cum in your mouth.

You should know that when a man is ejaculating the head of his penis is going to swell quite a bit in your mouth. This is going to be perceptible right before he cums. This is a physical tip from his body to get ready. You should be waiting and looking for this tip. When you feel that, you know that he is about to ejaculate and again you can make sure only the tip is in your mouth. At this point keep up your hand motion and you will ensure a perfectly controlled release into your mouth.
Now, as for your mouth itself, with only the tip of his penis in your mouth (no deep throating at this point) you are really in control of how he ejaculates. What you can do is tilt your forehead down as you angle the opening of his penis directly onto your tongue. You can even cup your tongue to receive the semen. This will form a perfect receptacle for the semen to collect and will make sure that none winds up in your throat, at the same time the blowjob completes in a smooth, natural finish.

Now all you need to do is figure out what to do with that semen.

What To Do With That Semen

Well, the old adage of spit or swallow really illustrates the two choices that you face when a man is cumming in your mouth. Those are your two options really. However, I do have a few words to add to the discussion.

First, if you really just can't stand semen in your mouth, one thing you can do is this. When you have angled your forehead down and he is cumming onto your tongue, you can open your mouth. What will happen at this point, is that as the semen is released, it will run right down your tongue onto his balls. This is the fastest way to get it out of your mouth. Also, you won't have to stop any oral pleasuring to do this.

If this is to much coordination, you can hold the semen in your mouth and then elegantly spit it into a towel that you cleverly placed next to the bed. If you think you can't hold semen in your mouth, you are wrong. Just go gargle some water and you will realize how much you are in control of swallowing after all.

If you do decide to swallow, it is really not bad. I have tasted semen plenty of times and the flavor is really quite benign. If you do decide to swallow just do it quickly and I would recommend a quick swig of water as well. You should always have water and a towel next to the bed whenever there is wild oral sex going on. It's just best to be prepared.

So those are your options as far as semen in the mouth is concerned.

If You Really Just Can't Do Semen In The Mouth

Some people just cannot deal with semen in their mouth. They just can't. Well if this is the case, it is much better to use one of these tricks I am about to show you than it is to vomit or have a panic attack. Trust me, these are better.

The first trick is to use a blowjob as just foreplay. This is when you use your mouth to simply get him excited enough to engage in intercourse. He can then orgasm inside of you and the whole issue of semen in the mouth is sidestepped. This is really a great tip. Like I've said, a blowjob without orgasm as a means of foreplay is a great way to get him excited and often cumming inside someone during intercourse is just as good if not better than cumming in their mouth. It's the old bait and switch and he and his cock will never complain. Trust me.

The next option you have is to manually stroke his penis with your hand until he orgasms. The way I see it, if you choose this technique, you have two options. The first is that you have him cum on you. Many men find this very arousing. I am not one to cum on a woman's face. Honestly I have never gotten the appeal of that, but many men like this. Cumming on a woman's breasts are also very popular. There is an element of domination and territory marking here that definitely appeals to a man's mind (even on a subconscious level).

If you really can't deal with semen in your mouth, just follow one of the these moves listed in this section and you should be just fine. Remember, you can also always work your way up to semen in the mouth. This has been the case for me with women in my life, and often their attitudes change over time. Just do what works for you.

Oral Sex Foreplay

At this point, I have discussed in detail the basic blowjob. You should think of the basic blowjob as the technique that you use when it is time to make a man orgasm. This should not take long. A well rythmed basic blowjob should have little trouble making a man cum in less than five minutes or so. In some cases, this is exactly what you want. However, I would strongly encourage you, as you work to become an expert on oral sex, to take your time with a blowjob. Although there is work involved, it should not be a chore. Instead, it should be play between two concerning adults who care for each other. It should be fun. There should be teasing. There should be slow licking and gentle kissing. You should work up to the basic blowjob slowly. Don't rush. There should be as much foreplay to an act of oral sex as there is to an act of intercourse. If you just get in there and bang it out, you are missing out on so much of the magic, fun and passion.

I am not going to give you a play by play method for foreplay. That would defeat the whole point. All that I will say is that you should work to give slow, soft attention to every part of his bikini zone. Only when you feel he is good and relaxed and at the same time thoroughly aroused, then should you start to actually stimulate him to orgasm with the basic blowjob technique.

Deep Throating

So much is made of deep throating these days. The adult film industry and popular culture make this sexual act out to be the greatest thing in the oral sex realm. Well, let me tell you, it's all crap. You most definitely do not need to be able to deep throat to give an amazing blowjob. Actually, since we know that the vast majority of a penis' nerves are at the very tip, you know that you don't stimulate anything extra by shoving the whole thing down your throat. Sure, it is a nice trick if you can do it, however, it is not at all necessary. The steps listed in the basic blowjob section are all that is required. So, if you gag, or are intimidated by deep throating, don't give it a second thought. Stick to the basics and master those. I'm confident the men in your life will not even notice because you will already be an amazing cocksucker. Trust me.

You Can Get Good & Rough

One thing that I want to make clear to all you ladies is that the penis is tough. It is really designed to be a battering ram. A lot of women seem to be very cautious about hurting a man's cock. They look at a penis through the lens of their pussies, which by comparison, are delicate and sensitive. Don't worry. You can spank, bite, nibble, pinch and vigorously stroke his cock all you want.
Now, there is one area that you need to be delicate with and that is his balls. These are sensitive and can be harmed if you are not careful. We will talk more about his balls and just what you are supposed to do with them in a bit.

Eye Contact

A lot of women do not understand the effect and connection that can be created when you make eye contact during a blowjob. Again, this is simply a result of the differences between men and women. Women, when they are getting their pussies eaten, tend to focus on the physical sensation. They do not watch the man (or woman) between their thighs intently. For them, the show is secondary. This is definitely not the case for men.

Men very much want to watch you suck their cocks. They will be watching you intently and they will be enjoying what they see. You can add to that with eye contact. Looking him intently in the eyes while he watches his cock slide into your mouth will only heighten his pleasure. It will say that you are turned on by what you are doing and that his pleasure is important to you. A woman looking into the eyes of the man who she is blowing is not a woman who is doing him a favor, but is a woman very much enjoying the sexual act she is performing. This is incredibly arousing to men. Eye contact also has the effect of creating connection between the couple. By looking him in the face, you will be able to see his reactions of pleasure. This is a great way to learn through direct observation what he enjoys.

Non-Goal Oriented Blowjobs

When I described the basic blowjob in an earlier part of this work, I was outlining a series of steps that are guaranteed to make the man in your life cum, and cum quickly, through your oral loving. The entire process should not take more than a few minutes of vigorous suck/stroking. This might be perfect for those quickie blowjobs when you duck into the ladies room at a concert or off the trail on a hike. However, if that were all that I taught you, I would be doing you quite a disservice.

There is a lot more to blowjobs than just a basic quickie. Men and women share a love of attention and the thought of their lover's hands, mouth and body. Ask yourself a question. When a partner of yours is eating your pussy, do you want them to charge right for your clitoris and begin vigorously stimulating it? I will assume you said no. Well, men are no different. That's where non-goal oriented oral sex comes in. If the basic blowjob provides you with the fundamentals of fellatio skills, this concept is where you add the passion, playfulness and fun.

There is not a step by step playbook for this part of oral sex. What unfolds between two lovers in the middle of this act is deeply personal and will be driven by their collective souls, spirits, hearts and passions. I can't tell you what to do. However, I can tell you how to know what to do.

Imagine having your lover lie on the bed again like when I told you how to give the basic blowjob. His head is at the top of the bed and you are facing him at the foot. Imagine that you trade places. How would you want your lover to touch you? Where would you like them to kiss, lick, suck nibble or caress? How would you like them to touch you? Where would you like attention? What would you like them to whisper in your ear? How would you want them to look at you while the kissed your most intimate and sensitive places? This is how you should touch him. Take your time. Explore his body and savor his reactions to your touch and kiss. Take your time. His excitement and arousal will only build. As a good measure of his arousal, look for the tell tale signs of pre-cum at the tip of his penis.

Two bits of advice that I will offer you however, are to always pay attention to his cock. No matter how the two of you contort your bodies, you should somehow always be paying attention to his penis. Men tend to be more impatient than women, and can frustrate. However, if you are always paying attention to his cock, this shouldn't happen. He will be wondering what you are going to do next. Also, don't be afraid to tell him your intentions. Whispering "I'm going to make you cum in my mouth." will most certainly communicate your intentions to pleasure him orally in no uncertain terms. Men will appreciate the directness, even if you take your time in getting there.

The Blowjob As Foreplay

Where a woman is concerned, you cannot stop eating her pussy and switch to intercourse only for her to cum moments later. It just doesn't work that way. However, the same is not true at all with the blowjob. You can suck your man until he is moments away from cumming, stop, and slip it inside you only for him to happily pump himself to orgasm and fuck you silly in the process. In fact, this is often a lot of fun.

What I am really saying here is that blowjobs are not simply a suck him until he cums or don't put your mouth anywhere near his cock problem. There is a wide range of possibilities here and you and he will have a lot of fun exploring them. Blowjobs can most definitely be a very, very fun bit of foreplay. You would be silly to ignore that facet of the blowjob in your sex life.

Spirit Of 69

Men are much more visually oriented than women and focus a great deal on what they see to turn them on. Knowing this, you should not be surprised that men are big fans of the "69" position. You can most definitely incorporate this into your oral sex games.

To do this, you should have your gentleman friend lie on the bed. Have his head about two feet from the top. If this means his legs dangle off the end of the bed, so be it. Now, straddle his face so you are looking at his feet. Once you have done this, you can then place his penis in his mouth and begin your blowjob.

If you choose to play with 69, there are a few things that you should know. First, most women are going to have trouble orgasming from anything he is going to be doing down there. The coordination required to keep the blowjob going is going to distract most women. Also, the body positioning of the 69 is really just not good for pussy eating. He is coming at her clitoris the wrong way to properly stimulate it. If you do 69, you should really just consider it adding another element (i.e. Your pussy right in his face) to the blowjob. This is still about his pleasure at this point. Of course, his mouth on your pussy may be more than enough to get you wet and constitutes a very good bit of foreplay.

If you choose to blow him to orgasm in the 69 position, you are also going to need to rethink your mouth positioning when he orgasms. It is still possible to direct the ejaculation onto your tongue, but you are going to need to stretch your neck a bit. Also, you may not be able to hear him call out before he orgasms. He may be muffled by your thighs and pussy. That's OK too. Generally as he approaches orgasm, he will stop licking your pussy. He will be too distracted. Take this as your cue.

The Quickie Blowjob

Like I have said, the basic blow job technique that was outlined earlier in this work, should be more than capable of bringing a man to orgasm in just a few short minutes. Start to finish. A man can also be ready willing and able for oral sex in just a few minutes. With the design of male attire he can also have his penis out in no time. These three facts make possible the quickie blowjob.

The quickie blowjob is when a couple decides to engage in oral sex while out and about. This can happen any number of places. Maybe they duck into an elevator or a public restroom together. Perhaps a deserted stairwell. Maybe on a hiking trail.

This can be a fun, naughty way for two people to engage in sex that can add a lot of excitement to a relationship. This is generally considerably more possible than eating a woman's pussy on the go (although it can be done) and is something that you should discuss with your lover. For many, the thrill of getting caught only adds to the fun!

Practice Makes Perfect

A while ago, a woman and I were sitting in a restaurant having lunch. She is a friend of mine and we were having a lively conversation. We talked about our lives and what we were up to and what was going on. Well, of course, I discussed this project with her. There are no secrets between the two of us. She laughed, and like most women when I told them about this work, started volunteering tips, tricks and advice. A lot of it wasn't new. However, she did tell me a pretty amusing story that I think is relevant to our discussion.

Apparently, she did not lose her virginity until she was 19. Until that time she had been a bit prudish. Like so many young women, her freshman year at college had been a bit of a turning point. She told me that she needed to learn how to give a blowjob and was simply mortified at the idea of seeming inexperienced (which she was) when the time came for her to get to work.

Well, she came up with a plan. She went out and bought herself a realistic dildo (veins and everything) and her and her roommate spent a fair amount of time getting comfortable with a cock shaped object in their mouths. She said she even learned to deep throat with it!

Now, for me, this sort of thing had been akin to the slumber party sleepover pillow fight. I had just assumed that it was a figment of our collective imaginations. To find myself face to face with a woman who was confirming that college coeds stay up late learning to give blowjobs together was more than appealing. However, I realized that she had brought up an, until then, ignored point.
If you want to get good at something and not seem inexperienced (a common enough fear for all of us), you need to practice. Why would blowjobs be any different? Why would we expect perfection right out of the gate?

You can find this experience in only one of two ways. Find a partner who is not going to mind working up your cock sucking expertise, or you can find a cock shaped object and practice on your own. If you don't feel comfortable buying a realistic dildo (although you can do this virtually anonymously on the internet), try the vegetable section of your local grocery store. I'm thinking carrot.

You Are In Control – Enjoy It

One thing that anyone planning to suck a cock should understand, is that they are most definitely in control. When you have a man's cock in your mouth, he is completely at your mercy. You control whether or not he will be happy or sad, and whether or not he will receive the one thing he wants most in the world – to orgasm in your mouth. Everything else fades into the background. He would do anything, say anything to please you to finish. You may be on your knees, but you are the one in charge. Often, you can use this to heighten the blowjob and your sense of control. Feel free to tease him. Keep him guessing as to your intentions. He is putty i your hands here, if nowhere else. You can and should enjoy the control as much as you do the pleasure you are giving him.

"It Turns Me On When You Tell Me What To Do"

A lot of men have trouble discussing what they like during sex. They are happy to stick it in, move it around a bit until they cum. However, that doesn't tell you anything about what turns them on and what they enjoy from you and doing to you. This is a huge roadblock to giving a good blowjob. You are going to need to get them to talk to you and tell them what they like.

The best way to do that is to use a little psychology. Men want their women to be turned on by them. This is important to them. They want you to enjoy sex. So what you do is this. You tell them that you are going to give them a blowjob, and you want them to tell you what to do. You tell them that they are the boss and it turns you on for them to boss you around. Most men will only be too happy to oblige. In bossing you around, they are really telling you what they enjoy and they are having you do it. In all reality, they are giving you a one on one class on how to give them a tailor made, perfect blowjob.

Dealing With A Limp Cock

In my sex life I have dealt with a limp cock plenty of times. You need to not be intimidated by this. It is entirely possible that you are getting hot in heavy in the back of a car in the parking lot of some mall, you pull down his pants with the intention of taking the head of his hard cock in your mouth, only to find that things are not especially hard down there. To some women, this is going to be a huge ego hit and they may not recover from it.

This doesn't need to be the case. A limp cock is by no means an insult or a sign that the man is not into what is happening. When you first start making out, does your pussy immediately become wet? No, this can take time and direct stimulation. Well a penis is no different. It just needs a little direct attention and it will be rock hard in no time. Actually, with a penis, it's very easy. Just take the whole limp thing and put it in your mouth. Play with it with your tongue while you gently cup his balls and it will be hard in no time. In fact, you will actually feel it getting hard in your mouth as you do this. In no time, he will have a full fledged erection that will be already lubed with your saliva and you can commence the wonderful blowjob you had planned on.

The Don't Call It A BlowJOB For Nothing

Anyone who cares about the pleasure of their partner enough to engage in oral sex, needs to be able to come to grips with the fact there may be some discomfort. Let's just put it on the table and talk about it. When I am eating a woman's pussy this is definitely the case. My neck can get stiff, my wrist may get tired, my jaw can get sore. Maybe I'm under the covers and its getting pretty hot and sweaty down there. Why should it be any different when I give a blowjob?

In my conversations with the ladies in my life concerning the act of sucking a man's cock, they have reported many of the same occurrences. Their jaws and wrists get tired and their necks get sore. So what? When you run a marathon, you know you are going to be sore when you're done. However, it feels absolutely wonderful when you finish. Well, the same is true for oral sex. Sure there may be some (mild at worst) discomfort along the way, but in the end, that all means nothing when you feel your lovers body tense in pleasure and relax at release. You feel great at the pure act of giving them pleasure and the sense of accomplishment. So when you're in there, on your knees, cock in your mouth and you start feeling those muscles beginning to ache, ignore it. Focus on your lover and their pleasure. In the end, you will find it worthwhile.

Sometimes It Just Ain't Gonna Happen...It's OK

I said this in my work on pussy eating and I would by a bit of a hypocrite if I did not include the same message in this work. So here goes. Sometimes you can suck his cock all you want and do it perfectly, just to have him not reach orgasm. It's OK. Don't beat yourself up. Orgasms and human sexuality can be a little tricky. This is art, not science. Remember that.
Lot's of things can cause this. Maybe his head isn't in the right place. Maybe he had a rough day at work. Maybe you came home horny, just after he had masturbated (been there done that) and he just won't fess up. No matter how good that blowjob is, you're not going to make him cum two minutes later.

You can't go through life expecting everything to be perfect. It definitely should not be read that you did something wrong, he doesn't find you attractive, or that you should give up on oral sex as a whole. That would just be silly. Instead, talk about it. Put it out on the open and reassure each other about your feelings. Be patient and understanding That is the healthy adult thing to do. That and try giving him a blowjob tomorrow just for good measure. I very much doubt he will argue with you.

What's Good For The Goose

I am a big believer in equality. Equality in a relationship along with a give and take spirit of compromise is one of the keys to a long lasting, supportive, mutually beneficial, and healthy relationship. That concept applies to the bedroom as much as it does to any facet of your relationship. If you are reading this book, you are interested in pleasing your lover. It is as pleasurable to me to give oral sex as it is to receive it. However, I sure as hell like to get it. If you are going to all this trouble to learn to please your lover, it is my sincere hope that they are just as interested in pleasing you orally.

After reading this book, I am sure that you will be excited to go out and try all that I have taught you. At the same time, I hope that you will insist, if need be, on your lover getting down on their knees and pleasuring you as well. Never forget what's good for the goose is good for the gander.

In Conclusion

Thank you for reading this work. At this point, I am hopeful that you have learned much about how to pleasure a man orally. We have covered lots of techniques, tips and tricks in our little discussion. Now, it is up to you to put this all together and become a true blowjob goddess. I am sincerely hopeful that you will be able to do this. Always remember to enjoy yourself and to have fun. Also remember to keep the communication open and flowing. A blowjob is just like another sexual act. It is a partnership and requires the two of you to operate in harmony. Good luck and enjoy!

-C.W. Pollard

Printed in Great Britain
by Amazon.co.uk, Ltd.,
Marston Gate.